I dedicate this small piece of writing to my patients and my family, for which I am forever grateful.

Thank you!

Mark J. Stevens, DO

Transcendent Health by Dr. Mark J Stevens, DO

Preface

This short book is for both laypeople and professionals alike. I am imparting pearls and observations I have made over the years, and what I have found to be fundamental truths and patterns about health and wellness over the years, and wish to provide this information to anyone willing to listen and want to learn more about health and wellness. True, most of the ideas and topics I talk about, could be delved into much more detail, and the studies that have been done to corroborate these ideas could be included, however, I am trying to be as brief and concise as possible. Just like in an interview with a patient, I will not spend an entire day explaining and teaching a subject but will highlight the important parts that need to be heard, to lay the groundwork towards health and wellness. As a physician, my job is to first do no harm, and to find health in a person, not simply diagnose and treat diseases. My goal is to get patients better; to be healthy and well. There is a point in anyone's life where they are at the point of no return, but even then, tapping into the inner workings of our mind, body, and spirit can bring peace, acceptance, hope, and a sense of dignity in our lives. I hope that you find these passages meaningful and make sense in your daily life, and transcend your life to great heights. These passages may or may not extend your life, but hope to deepen it and make one's life more meaningful.   The references that I provide at the end will simply help you skim over the topics discussed, and provide more information/detail, and can provide even more links and references. The topics discussed can have books written about each topic alone, and the number of studies that have come out about many of these topics can be discussed and studied for years. To speed up this process I am integrating the systems to show a bigger picture.

Table of Contents

Keys to Health

Imagine living life healthy, happy, resilient and able to adapt to change and stress both mentally and physically. Imagine a life where you can transcend across the normalcy of illness and disease and come to a point where you are happy. Happiness is not just having money or being able to have everything you want necessarily, but to have your health (mentally, physically and spiritually), which you need. How can you be completely happy if you are not complete? Feeling complete is through the collection of key elements that transcend you to greater heights.

Life is worth living, and knowing key elements can help bring you back towards health. Your body is a complex network of interrelated parts that work together in synchrony and harmony to maintain health. Your body has self-healing mechanisms. When you get a cut, your body heals over time. These healing principles have been observed and talked about for centuries, and even in Osteopathic Medicine, the tenants say that the body has self-regulatory and self-healing mechanisms and that the structure (anatomy) and the function (physiology) are interconnected and intertwined. Without one, the other could not exist. Can you imagine plumbing in your house without the structures that hold and transfer water, or allow waste to pass through sewage passageways? And if a hose gets kinked, how does water pass through it differently or even at all depending on the severity of the kink. Your body acts just like this. The blood and lymphatic vessels, nerves, muscles, bones, etc., all have a system of passageways that must be free and clear to allow normal health and healing to exist. The right ingredients are important to allow your body to maintain homeostasis, which is a constant balance to maintain health (function and structure working together harmoniously). Much of what we know and think about health is a collection of these five pillars that hold you in harmony. These five pillars of health are the following: Nutrition, Sleep, Exercise, Spirituality, and Social Support. These pillars give your body wellbeing and the ability to stay resilient to both internal and external stressors that affect us daily.

Hundreds of thousands of years ago, different cultures around the world observed healthy and sick people, and many belief systems explained why someone got sick or stayed healthy. Even today, people of all backgrounds have deep routed beliefs as to why someone is sick and or healthy. There have been many misguided and down-right false belief systems that still cloud our healthcare system today, that rely upon biased information or opinions of people that may not know the truth, nor want to espouse the truth because it may prevent them from making a profit, or keep them in a niche that holds those false beliefs to be true, and do not want to be exiled or punished by their profession and or management system at play. And often these truths about health care and medicine, in general, these days, by looking at morbidity and mortality rates linked directly from medical care (iatrogenic causes), you will see that orthodox medicine today is still stuck in the middle ages of belief systems. Take for example that medical providers are taught a doctrine of beliefs, such as about the myths about fats; that simply is not true, yet, many doctors, especially primary care doctors and other health professionals and health organizations measure their very patient outcomes based on surrogate markers (lab results that have their limits and faults), such as cholesterol levels, and makeup rules through opinions of professionals, who have no true evidence to support the treatments they espouse. Even though the truth is out there and there are many wise people and providers, many of these folks are not in mainstream medicine because of the very way our system is built and how it is run by health care insurance and management companies that dictate how patient care is given. We have a problem with our health care system that is full of confusing, and often misleading information.

Health literacy, which is how well a patient can navigate the health care system, is critical to surviving and dealing with the crazy system we have. Often literacy in general and knowing how to follow basic instructions are important, but even more important is teaching patients to better themselves through lifestyle changes, and doing motivational interviewing to activate and help motivate patients to take their health into their own hands, and take ownership of their health and wellness. Unfortunately, this is not the case in many outpatient clinics across the country. Today, just like a hundred years ago in America, there are dangerous medical treatments, and often increase death and disease (bloodletting to having patients ingest mercury salts back then, to prescribing statins, opiates, and other toxic drugs, to surgeries that were or now not necessary or caused more harm than good). Luckily, more and more data and evidence-based studies are showing that many of the believed treatments and ways to manage a disease are not appropriate, nor required for health. Evidence-based studies have decreased the aggressiveness and or the neglect of health problems/diseases, and over time has corroborated (strengthened) the philosophy and tenants of Osteopathic Medicine, and other forms of medicine across the globe that have been around for hundreds to thousands of years, that have helped to establish and maintain health and wellness (yoga, acupuncture, Ayurveda, Chinese and other herbal medicine treatments, meditation, tai chi, etc.).

Another problem in health care these days from my observations is that many patients also have unrealistic expectations and often demand treatments from the health care provider that are neither appropriate, nor safe often, and can lead to more problems down the road. The sad part is that health care providers will acquiesce and provide treatments that are dangerous to appease their patients. Studies have found that the happiest patients are often receiving subpar and substandard care. There must be a balance where patients have realistic expectations and know that medicine cannot cure, but rather treat illnesses and diseases. And often what patients want is not accessible in a doctor's office: Health. Health comes from within and it must be tapped into through the five pillars of health. Relying on natural, often safer ways to help facilitate and enhance health is the key, not necessarily on a health system that is often broken, and misleading. Health care is important and can be used appropriately for many conditions, which does save lives, but there is always a balance. The extremes of anything are not good.

To feel whole and well, and to have health, and to meet these 5 pillars of health, we must meet Maslow's hierarchy of needs which are very basic for health and wellness as well. We cannot be at the bottom of the pyramid at survival mode (poverty struck/low income/poor working-class/students/children), and rely on a health system ran by the government (Medicaid/Medicare/Indian Health Services), to bring people to health. Health is a multi-faceted phenomenon that requires basic requirements for the foundation of health to even occur. It almost seems like a cyclic process, how one can sustain the basic needs of shelter, food, safety, etc. If one is not healthy enough to work and or provide for themselves with the basics.

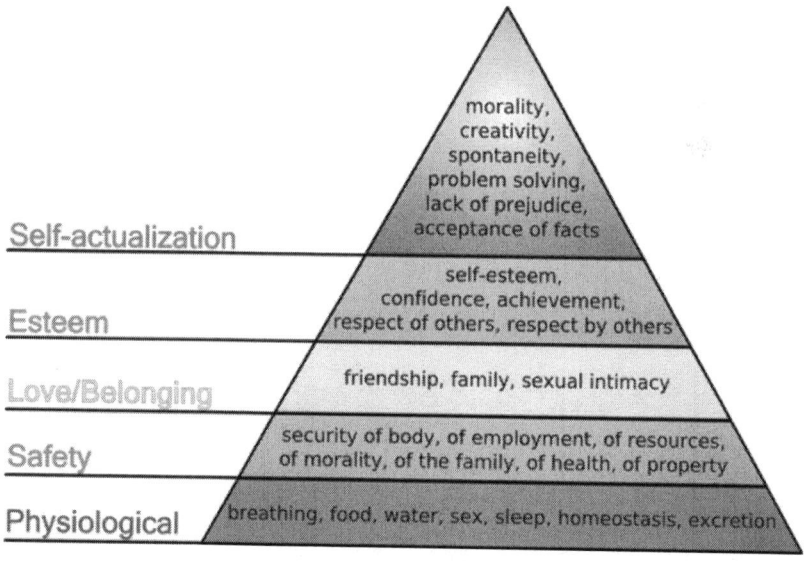

Maslow's Hierarchy of Need

Often people can get stuck in ruts because they fall into a cyclic process of illness and disease because they cannot break the cycle and do not know how to get out of it. Once injuries or problems go on for too long or are severe enough this is going to take a toll on the body and the mind and will reduce one's ability to be resilient and get out of the rut. This book is not intended to provide a path to monetary prosperity, nor cure every one of their mental and physical illnesses; however, this book is designed to help one tap into their body's healing mechanisms to help bring back health.

Unlike allopathic medicine (M.D.s), osteopathic medicine (D.O.s) have a philosophy built into our health model that espouses that we should bring people back towards health, and not solely focus on disease. A disease is an entity of or a collection of dysfunctional problems that do not allow the normal anatomy and physiology to work at its pinnacle. Anyone can find disease and illness, but a great physician and or person of healing can find health in a person and bring it back. Often prevention and lifestyle changes are the most important factors, and it relies on education and knowledge of core principles of health.

For the mind, body, and spirit to be complete, we must have certain keystone elements. We will go into further detail into each area and paint a picture in broad strokes and go into further detail based on my observations.

Osteopathic Tenants

To understand health and wellness, reflecting on Dr. A. T. Still's original four key principles (written in 1874) that give the foundation to understanding and helping patients come back towards health and to maintain health. These four principles are the following:

1. The body is a unit, and a person is a unit made up of body, mind, and spirit.

2. The body can self-regulate, self-heal, and maintain health.

3. Structure (anatomy) and function (physiology) are interrelated and interconnected and are reciprocal to one another.

4. Rational treatment is based on the understanding of these above-aforementioned principles. In broad strokes understanding these principles allows for the development and execution of sound diagnostic and treatment plans that are individualized/personalized to each person.

Often when looking at individuals, we see that no one is cookie cutter. Everyone is special in their own right, and has different needs and wants, and often something that may be good for one person, may not be good for another. However, saying that, there are core principles that follow basic laws of nature that without these key elements, a person's health cannot be maintained. Medical treatment should be tailored and individualized, and should not be overbearing to an individual, a family and or society as a whole. Medical treatment should be kept simple, easy to understand, and left between the provider and the patient. That is why I believe insurance companies and bureaucrats should stay out of medicine. They often try to dictate and run medicine from misguided and fallacious points of view/ideas that do not focus necessarily on ways to keep patients healthy. Insurance companies are designed to take your money and run. They are good at denying claims and care so that they can make a profit. They rely on fear, and of patients not knowing the truth about health and wellness. Insurance should be designed for catastrophic events only (Inpatient hospital care is very expensive, and can leave one or one's family in a lot of debt, if not for insurance), not outpatient medical care.

Rational treatment plans should focus on how to bring a patient back to health and keep that person healthy. Rational treatment should first "Do No Harm", and be effective and efficient. Often the best medicine is a healthy lifestyle, which includes the five pillars of health.

Just like plumbing or electrical work, an astute physician and or healer should observe and look for dysfunctions that would further cause problems that would obstruct, hinder, or decrease the normal function of the body. If a pipe is kinked, just like a blood vessel, the flow is decreased or impeded, where fluids cannot move freely anymore and cause stasis. This means that normal movement is not occurring as it should and hinders normal function, thus this is a dysfunction.

Using the basic tenants of Osteopathy, the provider has three objectives to achieve with manipulation of the body:

1. Remove any obstructions or impingements of the structures, enhancing the normal fluid flow of the nerves, blood vessels, and lymphatic channels to allow for self-regulatory maintenance.

2. Improve upon and or reestablish normal range of motion of joints and muscle/fascial tissues to their most functional and ideal state.

3. Balance the autonomic nerve flow by either stimulating and or removing impingements and irritation of the parasympathetic and sympathetic nerve tissues that are near the spine and along the cranium, which affect self-regulatory mechanisms and healing. These principles are taught and actively used in Osteopathic Medical schools, and Osteopathic physicians who choose to continue practicing Osteopathic Manipulative Medicine and Treatment (OMM/OMT) and Neuromusculoskeletal Medicine (NMM).

Thus relieving impediments and impingements of the structure (anatomy) allow for normal function (physiology). Anatomy and physiology are intertwined, and thus the function affects the structure, just as the structure affects the function. Normal maintenance and health ensue when the structure and the function work together harmoniously.

Stress, Health, and Disease

The body, just like a bridge or any other structure for that matter, can become weakened by stress. Often we think of mechanical stressors, but in living bodies, such as ours, and other living creatures, we can have many different forms of stress that may or may not be as obvious as trauma or some structural change. For example, mental stress, internal and external stressors can have a deep impact on our overall wellbeing and thus our health (e.g. neglect, extreme temperatures, malnutrition, mental and physical abuse, inadequate water intake, oxidative stress, light and sound injuries, etc.)

Over and over again, more and more data have shown the negative repercussions of long-term stress. Acute stress may be a good thing, for example, it may save us from a wild bear chasing us when we are walking in the forest and need to find a way to survive. The fight or flight responses have basic survival instincts build into our system, which is primarily unconscious and harbor deeper systems that are not readily available to our conscious mind. Just like some stressors, anxiety is a form of stress that is often a sign from the Universe that something in our lives needs to changes, either our environment, ourselves, and if we cannot change our environment or ourselves, we then must learn to cope and deal with these stressors in a way that allows us to survive and move on. When our body and mind cannot maintain balance, and our window of dysfunction is breached, the system begins to fail. Chronic, ongoing stress is called allostatic load, and over time, if the stress is not removed, it will cause marked dysfunction, eventual catastrophe (disease) and even death. Death is the outcome when the body can no longer maintain its basic normal functions and the system shuts down completely.

Health then is the vital outcome of the entire system working together harmoniously to maintain a life that maximizes the integration of mind, body, and spirit. We all have a window of dysfunction that our bodies can continue to maintain health and to function, and we cope and deal with stressors on a day to day basis. We can do this because just like in chemistry with buffer systems, our body is one great buffer system that allows for stressors to be mitigated. Disease by then is simply the inability of the body to maintain that normal balance and the systems are not working harmoniously anymore. The life force is being choked. For example, when little blood vessels, such as capillaries and or arterioles, and even arteries that carry life-sustaining blood with oxygen and nutrients are shut off or the flow is reduced due to obstructions, this can cause localized areas of ischemia (lack of oxygen to tissues/cells), which can cause a cascade of events leading to further tissue and cell injury, such as a heart attack, which then affects the ability of the heart to beat properly, and or pump blood efficiently. So a small change can have a big impact.

The best medicine is to try to maintain health, but people that have a disease can also be brought back to health, but finding ways to help facilitate healing and health, by removing those impediments that cause and or lead to disease. The role of the physician should not be to simply focus on disease but to focus on health and bringing patients back towards health through their inner life force system. Part of bringing people back towards health is through and maintaining the key elements of health, which include nutrition, sleep, spirituality, exercise, social supports, and other mechanisms to help give one resiliency to stressors both internally and externally.

Keystone Elements

Keystone elements are just that, they are critical to life function and are the key to success. Without these elements that system fails. People can and will argue many things are keystone elements. I will talk about the five pillars of your health that are part of the Keystone network. From each of these pillars, I will note what is keystone about each element. Just like a well-oiled machine that works effortlessly, it takes an integrated system to work harmoniously.

Nutrition

 Nutrition is one of the primary key elements of health. And within nutrition, there are a lot of myths and confusion, often foods pushed by large corporations and or pushed by people and companies that have an interest in solely making money, and have no interest in one's actual health. Often people that make foods for the sole interest of making a profit, and lobby government to push for fake, modified, processed and manipulated foods for their self-interest and profit, misguiding and manipulating the health care system is one of the basic reasons I have decided to write this book.   I spend a lot of time with my patients, talking about nutrition.

 Without nutrition, many of the other factors do not matter, and your body cannot do what it needs to do, to maintain health. How can you manage basic ion channels that help muscles contract, and nerves to send pulses without magnesium, for example? Magnesium is a keystone nutritional element that is required for over 300 metabolic processes in your body, activating and running enzymes and ion channels that are critical for normal function. Studies have shown that if one eats a well-balanced diet, such as the Mediterranean diet, many basic vitamins become obsolete. However, most patients that I encounter do not eat a well-balanced diet, and often they do not know that a daily multivitamin still does not contain enough of the keystone nutritional elements required for basic functioning.

As a physician, who trained in Maine, I saw a lot of nutritional deficiencies, and the most common that I see over and over again is the following: Vitamin D deficiency, and low magnesium. These truly are keystone nutritional elements unlike any other because without these elements they cause a broad spectrum of problems and manifestation of diseases that may not seem so obvious.

Low magnesium (hypomagnesemia), affects everything in the body. Manifestations of low magnesium include the following: Migraine headaches, seizures, poor wound healing, anxiety/depression, muscle cramping, muscle aches and pains, palpitations, dizziness, immune dysfunction, weakness, fatigue, thyroid dysfunction, metabolic dysfunction, hypogonadism (decreased sex hormones), osteoporosis, acne, increased risk of infections, increased pain, decreased ability to cope and deal with stress, etc. The list goes on and on because it is so critical for so many things in the body. When I worked in the Emergency room and was a hospitalist managing patient care in the hospital, I had to make sure that the patient's magnesium level was normal before I could even consider replacing their other electrolytes such as potassium, sodium, calcium, etc. Without having normal magnesium levels, it does not matter how much potassium I try to replace, the body would not be able to use or manage the potassium.

Just as magnesium is critical for health, so is Vitamin D3. The active form of vitamin D, which is D3, is made by the kidneys. Making vitamin is a somewhat complex system that requires cholesterol molecules in the skin to be hit just right by enough adequate UVB light to change its structure to something slightly more soluble than the body will then bring to the liver and then the kidney through our blood system to make vitamin D.

Vitamin D is essential not only for calcium homeostasis, and the absorption of calcium from the intestines into the bloodstream, but also important for our immune system, and normal mental and physical functions. People that are low in vitamin D can present with fatigue, muscle aches, and pains, anxiety, seasonal affective disorder/depression, trouble coping and dealing with stress, poor wound healing, autoimmune disorders/diseases, increased pain, etc. White blood cells and other parts of our immune system cannot attack and kill viruses, bacteria, fungus or cancer without vitamin D.

Just like low magnesium, vitamin D deficiency and insufficiency can present with many of the same symptoms. Magnesium and vitamin D work together synergistically. When I was in Maine, doing my residency training, about 95% of the people I screened were low. Even in New Mexico, where I live now, I have seen about 75 to 80% of patients with vitamin D insufficiency and or deficiency. In Maine, we did many observational studies looking at vitamin D levels of nursing home residents, looking at their levels before and after treatment, and how long it takes to get back to normal. Most patients take about 3 months to get back to normal on high dose Vitamin D3 10,000 IU daily (250 micrograms – Note this is equivalent to 10 minutes of good quality sun exposure. In theory a person can make about 30,000 IU within 15-20 minutes of good quality sun exposure with their shirt off at the beach) or Vitamin D2 50,000 IU (1,250 micrograms) once weekly. Once levels are back to normal (above 30 ng/ml, ideally between 40-60 ng/ml) then one can take a maintenance dose, which is based on weight, which is 1,000 IU/50 lbs. of body weight/day, so about 3-5,000 IU daily for most adults.

I have found from personal experience and from many patients that I have treated over the years that the active form daily is better tolerated and has had better outcomes in terms of improvement in health and reduction in negative symptoms. If a patient has kidney disease, then they must receive the active form of vitamin D (vitamin D3), since their kidneys cannot make the active form. If one has liver disease, then the storage form of vitamin D may not be readily available for the kidneys to make the active form. The high dose 50,000 IU weekly is the liver form, also known as the storage form of vitamin D (vitamin D2). When a person is at the beach, let's say San Diego, and has their shirt off, and have good UVB light exposure to enough surface area of skin, they can make 30,000 IU within 15-20 minutes of sun exposure.

Magnesium, calcium, vitamins D3 and K2 are essential for calcium homeostasis, which is important for a wide array of metabolic processes in the body. Sure you can take calcium and vitamin K2 along with magnesium and vitamin D to help facilitate calcium homeostasis; however, taking calcium through food and or supplementation is not as critical as supplementing magnesium and vitamin D3. Vitamin K2 can be found in grass-fed/range free/cage-free animal fats/meats such as eggs, poultry, and beef. Vitamin K2 is essential for helping the body move/shuttle calcium from areas where it does not belong, such as the arteries, and puts it back in the bone and other places where it is normally needed/required. Most people require about 90 mcg per day of Vitamin K2. Generally, if one eats 2 eggs or eats either meat/poultry and or butter that has vitamin K2, theoretically one should not have to supplement necessarily.

Another caveat about calcium intake is that calcium generically binds to everything, so taking anything with calcium can potentially block the absorption of those nutrients and you will simply poop it out, to be frank. People will often say that they take vitamin D with their calcium, however, the dose of vitamin D in the calcium supplement is very low, and most of this will not get absorbed anyways because the calcium generically binds to it. One must take calcium and or eat foods with calcium separately and ideally 4 hours before and or after taking anything else.

Most adults need between 1,000 to 1,200 mg of calcium per day, which is equivalent to about 4 eight-ounce glasses of milk per day. Many people do not like milk, nor do they eat a lot of dairy food, and so supplementing is important. People that are on radical/extreme diets, or do not consume any animal products, should then supplement with B vitamins and fat-soluble vitamins since these are scarce or not as readily available in vegetables, fruits, beans/legumes. Balance again should be the key to success. When a person tries to stay on one side, going to extremes, it is like swinging on a pendulum, eventually, the pendulum will swing to the opposite side. This is pretty much true for anything in life.

The DASH Diet

The best well-studied diets that are evidence-based, and have shown significant outcomes in health, and reducing disease are the DASH diet study and studies on the Mediterranean diet. The DASH diet stands for the Dietary Approaches to Stop Hypertension, which is essentially a modified Mediterranean diet. They looked at thousands of people, and made little tweaks in their diet, and found that they could significantly reduce hypertension, along with other cardiac diseases/outcomes, reducing morbidity and mortality as endpoints (cardiac arrest, stroke, heart attacks, etc.)

The secret is eating clean, and removing processed foods, fake/synthetic additives and high amounts of salt from the diet. The DASH diet is essentially an avoidance diet, where one avoids all the toxins and chemicals in foods that can cause health problems. For example, Aspartame, which is an amino acid, a sweetener, is broken down primarily by the liver into formaldehyde and menthol, which are both toxic, and should be avoided. This is commonly found in diet sodas and gum/candy. There are many toxins and chemicals in foods that I could list, however, to keep it simple; I give most of my patients this following list of things to avoid:

- Avoid salt intake greater than 2,000 mg per day (this is usually a teaspoon of salt per day)

- Avoid Aspartame and other synthetic/amino acid sweeteners

- Avoid processed and canned foods that contain a lot of salt and sugar

- Avoid concentrated fruit juices due to the high sugar content

- Avoid MSG/Nitrates/Nitrites which are commonly found in cured meats. MSG is monosodium glutamate and acts as a super salt, and just like it is used to tenderize meat, it tenderizes your body and can increase the risk for headaches, seizures, and elevate blood pressures. It can also trigger Meniere's disease where people get severe ringing in their ears, with decreased hearing and episodes of dizziness. Nitrates and nitrites have been found to increase the risk for cancer, and can also affect blood pressures, and also cause dizziness. Often labels can be deceiving, where it will say hydrogenated or autolyzed yeast extract, which contains MSG. Soups, broths, Bouillon cubes, many Asian foods, etc. contain MSG.

- Avoid GMO/genetically modified corn and wheat products that contain high-density proteins that can cause more inflammation in the gut and body.

- Avoid trans-fats. Frying most oils and cooking on high heat with mono and polyunsaturated fats can make trans-fats. Labels that say hydrogenated and or partially hydrogenated oils are also trans-fats. A classic example of trans-fat is margarine or anything that is synthetically converted from liquid oil to a sold fat.

• Avoid foods that contain corn syrup, high fructose corn syrup, maltodextrin, or other high-density sugars.

Often most people think of the macronutrients, which are sugars, protein and fat, which we need, but we also need the micronutrients that are in foods as well. For example, a strawberry contains over 70 different micronutrients. That is why processed foods are not good. They are depleted in most of the nutrients, which can cause malnutrition to ensue when one consumes primarily processed foods. Most of the micronutrients are removed; almost 98-99% of the micronutrients are gone by the time most foods are processed.

In regards to the macronutrients, I tell my patients the following: Sugars should primarily come from fruits and vegetables. Our protein should come from either animal sources that are clean, grass-fed/cage-free animals and or from soy/beans/legumes and certain grains. We need three types of fats, including saturated, monounsaturated and polyunsaturated fats. The best saturated fat is either grass-fed cow butter and or coconut oil (which is a medium-chain fatty acid that is found in Mother's milk). The best mono-unsaturated fat is olive oil and must be cooked with medium to low heat to not alter its structure, and most vegetable and soy oils must be avoided. The best poly-unsaturated fats are the Omega 3 fatty acids, which are found in eggs, avocados, and fish. Omega 6 and Omega 9 fatty acids are highly volatile and can become oxidized and become rancid very quickly, and can often cause more inflammation in the body. Omega 3 fatty acids are anti-inflammatory and good for the body as a whole.

Another great myth is the myth about all fats being bad for you. I often recommend my patients see the documentary, Fat Head by Tom Naughton, which debunks a lot of the myths about fats, and the documentary shows how many of these myths got started in the first place, and how many of these myths are so ingrained and taught in medicine and indoctrinated in mainstream media, etc. It was lobbyists, government officials and people of power that purposely mislead the public and lied about studies to gain profit shares in companies they owned or invested in that made bad foods, and some simply made bad decisions without truly looking at the evidence. Unfortunately, there have been many cases throughout the years where politicians and corrupt business people/lobbyists do not have the public interest at heart and often walk away with large amounts of money, using the public office as a medium to bribe and leverage business for their self- interest. Many prominent politicians over the years have made a lot of money by getting into office to exploit, take advantage of, lie and misguide the public, while making profits and funneling money into their bank accounts without the public knowing about it until recently.

Cholesterol

Cholesterol is a critical molecule in the body and is essential for life. Cholesterol is the precursor for many critical hormones in the body (cortisol, vitamin D, aldosterone, testosterone, and is important for basic normal cell membrane integrity. Often clinicians and scientists are confused and misguided. They see a relationship with something bad, and they think that cholesterol is bad. Just like when cardiologists and scientists saw that there was a relationship between calcium deposits in the arteries and with heart attacks, they decided that calcium was bad for people. But In fact, what we have is a problem with inflammation in the body, not calcium and or cholesterol.

Whenever you have inflammation, your body will take whatever it can from the bloodstream, which includes calcium and cholesterol. Inflammation is the underlying mechanism of laying down plaque, not cholesterol and or calcium. Laying down cholesterol and calcium deposits are a direct result of inflammation, not the other way around. Improving nutrition and activating your body's ability to reduce inflammation is essential to reducing plaque formation. This is done through the diet I discussed above and allowing your body to take care of the rest. The liver makes a very powerful anti-oxidant, called glutathione, and is activated with certain foods/nutrients and when the body is stressed.

The body also makes more cholesterol when the body/mind is stressed. Why do you ask? It is because cholesterol is the precursor to making stress hormones, such as cortisol. So when a person is stressed, cholesterol levels go up. It's that simple. I am not one of those doctors who jumped on the bandwagon and decided cholesterol was bad, and that everyone needed to be on a statin medication to block the production of cholesterol.

Cholesterol and lipid levels in the bloodstream tell me two things: Is the body stressed, and is this person taking in too many simple carbohydrates (sugars) and or do they have high blood sugars. When a person consumes or eats a lot of sugars or if they have markedly elevated blood sugars, the body converts those sugars into triglycerides. That is why when triglycerides rise it is an indication that a person may also be developing diabetes and or pre-diabetes. Treating pre-diabetes and even diabetes first-line is still and will always be changing diet and making lifestyle changes first. Taking statins can cause more problems, and often the risk of taking statins includes muscle and liver break down, hypogonadism, electrolyte imbalances, and vitamin D deficiency, etc.

Most of our chronic diseases are brought on by lifestyle choices that we make (consciously and or unconsciously) or exposed to elements that affect our health. Some things we may simply not know about as an exposure. Many things in the environment can cause problems and even lead to cancer and other ailments that we may not necessarily have control over. But we can maximize what we have control of to the best of our abilities. When our immune system is healthy, it fights bacteria, viruses, fungus, and even cancer cells.

One last note about nutrition is also hydration. True you can overdo it, and you can definitely under do it. But most people that I see in the clinic are often dehydrated, meaning they are so low on water intake; that they can develop a myriad of problems, and are susceptible to getting kidney stones, kidney and bladder infections, can develop fatigue, palpitations (where the heart races very fast, and one is very aware of their heart beating fast), volume constriction, causing increased blood pressure, constipation, and increased stress response in the body. Just like the world is made up mostly of water, so is our body.

Sleep

Sleep is vital for health. Many diseases and disorders stem from a lack of good, restful sleep. There are a wide variety of causes of sleep troubles, as well as many remedies and recommendations, everything from diagnosing and treating sleeping disorders (insomnia) to actual sleep apnea (central/peripheral obstructive) in current medical practice, to behavioral health therapies (sleep hygiene), acupuncture, herbal supplements, meditation, breathing exercises, etc. Sleep is a very sensitive topic since it touches everyone in a very deep and meaningful way. Our dreams, our ability to decompress, heal and detoxify our minds and recharge our system is very important for the mind, body, spirit connection. The extremes have been seen with a person that cannot sleep at all; that is either due to an organic cause such as sleep apnea, to medication/drug-induced, causing extreme stress on the body. Over time, this stress, called allostatic load, comes crashing down, and the natural buffer system begins to fail, leading to diseases (obesity, hypertension, diabetes, cancer, etc.), to death.

Most sleep specialists agree that the minimum sleep required for good health is at least 6 hours of sleep, but ideally 7 to 8 hours of sleep for good health. Too little and too much sleep and lead to health problems. Also, another issue is that people that work at night or stay up at night, and sleep during the day, often have dysfunction with their sleep-wake cycles, and some folks can get shift work syndrome when they are constantly changing their schedule from night to day shifts.

Melatonin is one of the important regulatory hormones that are released in the brain to signal the body to go to sleep. This hormone can be easily suppressed by simply having blue light shining on the body and seen through the eyes; which triggers a cascade of events to stop the release of melatonin. Studies have shown that a chronic lack of melatonin over time, can lead to many chronic diseases, and increase the risk of heart attacks and strokes.

Sleep has its very own architecture and has a common pattern of waves that undulate into rapid eye movement sleep and deeper levels of sleep, that all work together in a pattern of resonance and vibrations.

When this architecture is disrupted a whole host of problems can ensue. Nearly 95% of patients that have fibromyalgia have interruptions with their REM sleep cycles. The REM (rapid eye movement) cycle comprises of the reticular activating system, that is related to awareness and being conscious while we are awake. We dream during our REM sleep cycles. In the brain and spinal cord, some pathways go up and down (brain into the spinal cord, and vice versa). The tethered, interconnected system of the reticular activating system, with the reticulospinal tracts, is responsible for attenuating and turning off pain signals from the spinal cord that travels up the brain. When our reticulospinal tracts are not regulated properly, pain signals can be amplified, causing marked pain and discomfort, leading to fibromyalgia aches and pains. By providing proper nutrition, and adequate sleep, patients with fibromyalgia can overcome their condition.

People that oversleep and under sleep can have a myriad of different problems; the more extreme the sleep dysfunction becomes, the more extreme the physiological, and mental problems that can occur.

Spirituality

Spirituality simply means what gives you meaning to your life. It could be religion; it could be your child or an idea of hope. Without hope, there is often no desire to live, nor continue and fight the good fight. When hope is gone, people that are depressed are most likely to commit suicide. Hope is an idea. Often fellow professors and colleagues would tell me not to give a false sense of hope. Hope however is an idea, it is a belief, and it is striving for something.

Hope is a powerful tool to mentally and physically striving to live and carry on. Hope, just like magnetic fields are invisible, and unexplainable, yet powerful and able to motivate and help us heal mentally, physically and spiritually. In spirit, just like our breath is necessary. Spirituality does not equal religion per se, but religion is one way to access spirituality and to provide hope.

Hope is not a tangible object, and that is why when you provide some inkling of hope, it is not false or true hope, it is simply an idea and or a belief that taps into our system to motivate us to live and take on the difficult tasks at hand. Without this critical piece of information, health and wellness cannot go on. Hope in a sense is like a computer program that is the glue that keeps us going. Atheists and agnostics are still spiritual; they still carry with them some kind of hope and have ideas of what gives their life meaning. All people can transcend their lives by having hope and spirituality.

Scientists have found many health benefits to spirituality, including daily practices of yoga, tai chi, meditation, prayer, breathing exercises. It helps people to ground themselves and regain their energy and focus. Many published works describe the importance of spirituality and health.

Our belief systems are tied into our wellbeing. When we give ourselves and others positive affirmations we transcend our health and wellness. Our vibrations increase and we are able to see past mental blocks, and let go of mental weights that keep us from being free. When we do the opposite, we become cold, our vibrations slow down, and depression and anxiety set in. When we are depressed, our hormones change, our ability to endure stress decreases and our thyroid function goes down. People can develop pseudo-dementia when they are severely depressed and anxious. The ability to turn this around is profound and possible. One only need to look at themselves and reflect and learn to love themselves for who they are and to let go of mental blocks and struggles that have no true bearing on who they really are. That is finding one's spirituality. To accept oneself for who they are and to understand and love themselves allows one to be compassionate for themselves and others. This in turn is spiritual nurturing for all living lifeforms.

Exercise

There are many ideas and opinions about the best way to exercise, and there have been many good evidence-based studies to support certain types of exercises to promote health and wellness. Fitness, as in science, is being fit to have children and carry on the legacy of the human race. Exercise helps with fitness, but also helps us to maintain our overall health and wellness. Exercise can be explored in much detail, and most people would agree that exercise is important for health.

Brisk walking (moderate-intensity) most days of the week for 30 minutes at a time is effective at maintaining a healthy weight and helps improve mood and overall well-being. When we exercise, our bodies release chemicals, such as serotonin, endorphins, enkephalins, cannabinoids, etc. These chemicals our bodies produce help improve our mood, decrease pain, and increase our stamina and ability to deal with stress. Strengthening exercises are just as important as aerobic exercises such as walking, running and swimming.

Core exercises that work along the abdominal, pelvic and lower back core are important for maintaining health and symmetry and reduce lower back pain, which includes planks and pelvic tilt techniques. Upper and lower strengthening exercises can be done 2-3 times per week, and brisk walking and other aerobic exercises should be done more frequently ideally. For both adults and older adults, the guidelines recommend 150 minutes of moderate-intensity aerobic activity or 75 minutes of vigorous-intensity aerobic activity and at least two days of muscle-strengthening activities per week.

Social Support

None of us can survive as a single unit without one another. Just like it takes hundreds of people to make a single pencil, to have a healthy well-balanced life, we require others in our lives, just like other people need us in their lives, either directly or indirectly. We are interconnected, whether we like it or not. And there have been documentaries, studies, and books written about social support and its relationship to health and wellness.

One documentary is the story of the Rosetans: a group of Italian immigrants living in Pennsylvania, who had less heart disease despite eating a similar diet, and had a similar lifestyle as the other people in surrounding towns, and it was directly linked to their strong social supports and family ties. This story was described in detail by Malcolm Gladwell in his book Outliers. There have been many examples shown, where the only difference was social supports, and the people that had the strongest social supports stayed healthier overall.

On a macro scale, we cannot live without the very Earth we live on, which supplies us with water, a medium to grow and raise food; a wide variety of challenges to help grow our minds and bodies, circadian rhythm of night and day, the energy that passes into and around us, helping us transcend our very lives. Even the heavens above and the ancient wisdom of our relationships with our selves and others help keep us healthy in many unexplainable ways.

On a microscale, just like our cells and all of its components must work together in a perfect symphony of vibration, movement, structure, and function influencing each other, our neighbors who are intimately close to us: Our Bio-flora in the gut have a strong overall effect and importance influence on our health. Studies have also shown that depending on what kind of bacteria reside in your gut, has major influences on our hormone balance, to affecting our stamina to making critical vitamins, e.g. vitamin K2, and several B vitamins just to name a few, to improving overall metabolic functioning, to influencing our immune system for better or worse. From macro social supports to micro supports, we are destined to have more or less health based on these support systems. Some supports we cannot necessarily choose (like our family), but we can choose our friends and the foods we eat that influence our gut.

Resiliency

Our bodies, our minds, and our very souls are put to the test, with both internal and external stressors that we must find ways to maintain balance and mitigate the negatives, and be able to withstand the storms of life. Resiliency is the ability to quickly recover from and overcome obstacles and stressors; a culmination of our five pillars of health.

Resiliency is a mental, physical, and spiritual tri-union that when perfectly balanced provides for maximum resiliency, health, and wellness. All people deal with stressors, and when those stressors become too much, and allostatic load can breach our walls and lower our abilities to stay healthy and well. We need stress in our lives to do well, but it must be balanced, and when the stress becomes toxic or too much, we can fall prey to its negative effects on our mind, body, and spirit. What comes to our defense is our ability to balance and maximize our five pillars: sleep, nutrition, exercise, spirituality, and social supports.

Inner peace and transcendence

The great feat of our lives is finding inner peace and transcendence. It is often thought to be of the highest level of our mind, body and spirit tri-union becoming whole. On the hierarchy of needs, this relationship and pinnacle of the higher levels of thought and feeling are transduced and elevated from within and with our relationship to the world and universe.

Our lives are shaped and influenced by energy and choices that are either within or without our control, and understanding that we live not as an island, but as part of a bigger picture, we are but a tree in a large forest, and to make sense that we are a part of a whole, we cannot live without having connections and meaning in our lives.

This is the truth about us and our world. We are all interconnected with each other and our world. True, all things must pass and the cycle of life continues, and our time is fleeting, it is the quality of time that we have and how we utilize and expand our lives to have a deeper meaning about ourselves and of others.

Summary

In Summary, one can transcend and tap into their health by activating and enhancing their lives through the five pillars of health. The mind, body, and spirit are interrelated and influence each other. Realizing the interconnectedness of ourselves with others and our universe gives us a deeper meaning. And as we provide our body, mind, and spirit with its basic keystone elements, we can transcend our health and wellness.

Biography

Dr. Stevens is Board Certified in Family Medicine and Osteopathic Manipulative Treatment through the American Osteopathic Board of Family Physicians. Dr. Stevens has a Bachelor's degree in Biochemistry from the University of New Mexico and received his D.O. degree from Touro University - Nevada. Dr. Stevens completed his Family Medicine and OMT training at Maine-Dartmouth Family Medicine Residency, while also completing over 200 hrs of Integrative Medicine training through the University of Arizona's Integrative Medicine Residency Program. Dr. Stevens emphasizes an integrative and individually based patient-centered approach, that focuses on health and wellness, which incorporates the five pillars of health, including proper sleep, good social supports, having meaning and or spirituality in one's life, proper diet and exercise.

References

McLeod S, Maslow's Hierarchy of Needs. Simply Psychology. 2007, updated 2016. https://www.simplypsychology.org/maslow.html

Still AT, Osteopathy: Research and Practice. Published by Restoration Editors New York, NY. Copyright 1910

Heinking, K, OMT Evidence Based Medicine. ACOFP 54th Annual Convention and Scientific Seminars 2017 http://www.acofp.org/ACOFPIMIS/Acofporg/PDFs/ACOFP17/handouts/FRIDAY/Fri_pm_200_Heinking,%20Kurt_OMT%20Evidence%20Based%20Medicine.pdf

Nelson, K, Osteopathic Distinctiveness. Somatic Dysfunction in Osteopathic Family Medicine. Copyright 2007 Lippincott Williams & Wilkins; Chapter 2:6-11

Institute of Medicine (US) Committee on Health and Behavior: Research, Practice, and Policy. Health and Behavior: The Interplay of Biological, Behavioral, and Societal Influences. Washington (DC): National Academies Press (US); 2001. 2, Biobehavioral Factors in Health and Disease. Available from: https://www.ncbi.nlm.nih.gov/books/NBK43737/

Arnetz B, Ekman R,Editors. Stress in Health and Disease. 2006. Wiley-VCH. Weinham 434p.

Logan JG, Barksdale DJ, Allostasis and Allostatic Load: Expanding the Discourse on Stress and Cardiovascular Disease. J Clin Nurs. 2008 Apr;17(7B):201-8

McEwen B, Allostasis and Allostatic Load: Implications for Neuropsychopharmacology. Neuropsychopharmacology. 2000;22:108-124

Vollmer WM, Sacks FM, Ard J, et al. Effects of diet and sodium intake on blood pressure: subgroup analysis of the DASH-Sodium trial. Ann Intern Med.2001 Dec 18;135(12):1019-28

Thacher T, Clarke B, Vitamin D insufficiency. Mayo Clin Proc. 2011 Jan; 86(1):50-60.

Rheaume-Bleue K, How Much Vitamin K2 Do We Need, and How Do We Get It? Vitamin K2 and the Calcium Paradox: How a Little-Known Vitamin Could Save Your Life. HarperCollins 2012; Chapter 3

Jahnen-Dechent W, Ketteler M, Magnesium Basics. Clin Kidney J. 2012 Feb;5(Suppl 1):i3-i14

Goldblatt J, Vitamin D Deficiency-Vitamin D Supplementation May Help Depression. Psychology Today;2011 Nov 14. https://www.psychologytoday.com/blog/the-breakthrough-depression-solution/201111/psychological-consequences-vitamin-d-deficiency

Mercola J, The Cholesterol Myth Has Been Busted – Yet Again. May 03,2017. https://articles.mercola.com/sites/articles/archive/2017/05/03/cholesterol-myth-busted.aspx

Naughton T, Fat Head. Documentary 2009.

Smith, Justin, $29 Billion Reasons to Lie about Cholesterol: Making Profit by Turning Healthy People into Patients. Copyright 2008 Matador.

Smith, Justin, 101 Causes of Heart Disease: High Cholesterol Isn't One of Them. Copyright 2016 Matador.

King P, Peacock I, Donnelly R, The UK Prospective Diabetes Study (UKPDS): clinical and therapeutic implications for type 2 diabetes. Br J Clin Pharmacol (BJCP).1999 Nov; 48(5):643-48.

Diabetes Prevention Program Research Group. Knowler WC, Fowler SE, Hamman RF, et al. 10-year follow-up of diabetes incidence and weight loss in the Diabetes Prevention Program Outcomes Study. Lancet. 2009 Nov 14;374(9702):1677–86.

Perreault L, Pan Q, Mather KJ, Watson KE, Hamman RF, Kahn SE, Diabetes Prevention Program Research Group Effect of regression from prediabetes to normal glucose regulation on long-term reduction in diabetes risk: results from the Diabetes Prevention Program Outcomes Study. Lancet. 2012 Jun 16;379(9833):2243–51.

Lindström J, Louheranta A, Mannelin M, et al. Finnish Diabetes Prevention Study Group The Finnish Diabetes Prevention Study (DPS): lifestyle intervention and 3-year results on diet and physical activity. Diabetes Care. 2003 Dec;26(12):3230–6.

Why Is Sleep Important? Sleep Deprivation and Deficiency. NHLBI/NIH/US Department of Health and Human Services. 2017 June. https://www.nhlbi.nih.gov/health/health-topics/topics/sdd/why

Spirituality and Health. American Academy of Family Physicians. 2017 May. https://familydoctor.org/spirituality-and-health/

Puchalski C, The role of spirituality in health care. Proc (Bayl Univ Med Cent). 2001 Oct;14(4):352-357

Ozby F, Johnson D, Dimoulas E, et al. Social Support and Resilience to Stress: From Neurobiology to Clinical Practice. Psychiatry (Egmont). 2007 May;4(5):35-40.

Meriwether R, Lee J, et al. Physical Activity Counseling. Am Fam Med. 2008 Apr 15;77(8):1129-1136

Lee PG, Jackson EA, Exercise Prescription in Older Adults. Am Fam Med. 2017 Apr 1;95(7):425-32

Gutkin, Cal. Outliers: extended families, better health outcomes - Why everyone should have a family doctor. Can Fam Physician. 2009 Jul; 55(7): 768.

Zolli, Andrew, Healy A. Resilience: Why Things Bounce Back. Free Press. 2012 (336pgs)

Shatte, Andrew, Reivich K. The Resilience Factor: 7 Keys to Finding Your Inner Strength and Overcoming Life's Hurdles. Harmony. 2013 (352 pgs).

Made in the USA
Middletown, DE
18 November 2025